All In

All In

The Mindset of Fitness

Bo Shappell and Daniella Land

DISCLAIMER: This book is designed to provide information and motivation to our readers. It is sold with the understanding that the authors are not engaged to render any type of psychological, medical, or any other kind of professional advice. This book is not intended as a substitute for the medical advice of physicians. The reader should regularly consult a physician in matters relating to his/her health and particularly with respect to any symptoms that may require diagnosis or medical attention. Before beginning any new exercise program, it is recommended that you seek medical advice from your personal physician. The content presented in this book is the sole opinion and expression of the authors. It is not intended to substitute for medical advice. Neither of the individual authors shall be liable for any physical, psychological, emotional, financial, or commercial damages, including, but not limited to, special, incidental, consequential or other damages.

ISBN-13: 9780692863589
ISBN-10: 0692863583

Table of Contents

Preface

A Note from Daniella

Sometimes the straight path isn't the best path. Sometimes the scenic route provides the most enjoyment. Writing this book has been a journey. I was not a fitness expert or an elite athlete when I started. I am someone who found success in an unusual, yet obvious place—someone who sees things differently.

Upon realizing this new mindset, I began to share it with my husband, Bo. As a physical education teacher, personal trainer, and coach, Bo is immersed in the fitness industry. He was intrigued and began adopting the approach detailed in this book.

Together we witnessed the counterproductive mindsets of his students and clients. We were continuously approached by people wanting to know our secret. What our regimens were. How we stayed motivated. To us it was so simple. We enjoyed it! Through those interactions, we began to see how our mindset contrasted theirs.

This book may surprise you. The journey to living and writing it certainly surprised Bo and me. So, why did we decide to write this book? Were we determined to tell the world how wrong its current method is? Did we feel it necessary to make others change? No, quite frankly at times the fear of that perception deterred us from writing this book. We do not need to change anyone or anything. We believe everyone is capable of following their own inner guidance toward the path in life that they desire. While we may be able to physically force someone to do something, the mind is different. We cannot force anyone's mind, or perspective, to change. It must occur from within. We are not here to judge anyone. Rather our intentions are to create something that resonates with us, to delight in sharing something beautiful, and to allow the seed I planted to continue to grow through, past, and beyond us. If you are drawn to this book, it is because there is something written here that you are calling into your life. That being said, I hope whatever you are looking for comes to you and that your eyes are open to see it. Enjoy!

One

Shift Your Focus

Let's Make Something Clear

This book is not an exercise or diet plan. It will not tell you what exercises to do, or rank which foods are best for your body.

You will need to take action. The difference, the critical differentiator of whether or not you will be successful, consistent, surpass challenges, and approach those actions with excitement, is your mindset training. The reason people "fail" is that they underestimate, or don't even consider, this factor.

The actions, the choices, the information related to fitness and nutrition will come easily to you once the tenets in this book are clearly understood, accepted, and established. You cannot ensure continual success by looking outside of yourself. You will never find lasting satisfaction there. Things change. Fads come and go, but the approach that breeds success can plant and grow within you.

If you allow it, this book will change how you perceive those things, and in turn the relationship you have with your body.

This book is a perspective changer—a guide to living all in.

The Right Approach

What you are about to read might seem like it has nothing to do with the rest of this book, but be assured; it does.

Imagine you have a friend who has difficulty finding and maintaining a romantic relationship. He claims he wants one, but the more conversations you share with him, the more apparent it becomes that he has a fear of commitment. He describes relationships as holding him back, being destined to fail, and taking away his freedom. All of this leads you to believe he is pushing away the very thing he supposedly desires.

How can he possibly have a successful relationship if he does not believe such a thing exists? How can he mentally overcome even a small disagreement with a romantic partner if he thinks the relationship is ultimately doomed to fail? How can he realize the joys of an intimate relationship if he views it as constricting his freedom? It is no wonder your friend is not successful. His mindset is holding him back because it is incompatible with his goals and desires. He needs to view and engage with relationships differently if he wants different results.

If you try telling your friend that his mindset is counterproductive, he will likely say you are wrong. To him, it is not his approach that needs to change. Instead, he blames circumstances and factors outside his control. He will only change once he realizes that he is internally conflicted and that his mindset doesn't support his goals.

So, what does this have to do with fitness? People take the same approach toward their bodies and healthy living that your fictional friend takes toward romantic relationships. They have a mindset that hinders them from achieving their wellness goals. It is not that they don't desire results—of course they do! Doesn't everyone want to look and feel healthy? Rather, their mindset is inharmonious with their aims. Because of this, they lack sufficient and sustainable motivation. However, just as your friend will have to stop making excuses and realize his approach needs to change, so do those struggling with fitness and healthy living.

Waiting on perfect circumstances breeds excuses. Perfection is a static notion, and life is not static. It is dynamic and evolving. Seeking the ideal diet and exercise plan, or waiting for the right amount of money and enough time, prevents people from moving forward. You will never start if you are waiting for the stars to align. Sometimes people do not see their excuses for what they are; instead, they see them as reality, which makes the situation unchangeable. If you require the ideal concoction of circumstances before you can experience progress and enjoyment, then you're making excuses. Rather than taking steps in the right direction and making the most of the situation, excuses leave us stuck with neither solution nor motivation. We must realize that it is not about perfection. It is about moving in the right direction. Only then can we move past excuses and establish a mindset that fosters continual success and enjoyment.

Too often, we focus only on physical results and try to force ourselves to follow whatever workout or diet someone else claims to be successful. We ride the waves of fads and trends, only to come crashing ashore once the excitement fades. The problem with that approach, is that we forget about our mindsets. This causes people to become discouraged, jump on and off the fitness bandwagon, over train and become injured, or, worst of all, not even try. We must be aware of our mental training if we really want to create lasting change. If you struggle, it likely is not your body's fault, but rather your mind's.

Your approach is not the only approach. Let that sink in. The ways you think and feel about working out, health, and fitness are not the only ways to think and feel about them. Most people do not reflect on this. They assume their views are absolute simply because they are the only ones they know. Those who struggle have counterproductive mindsets. They either don't believe success is possible for them, fear trying, lack motivation, or dread putting in the work. But here's the thing: people who live active and healthy lives do not see healthy living as work. To them, it is fun, natural, and invigorating. They crave it! This is not because they are already in shape. They have certainly faced challenges of their own. Ultimately, however, they have a different approach to healthy living. They are, what we refer to as, all in—mentally, emotionally, and physically committed.

Perhaps the idea of fitness seems grueling. Maybe you openly lack inspiration and energy. If so, your mindset is not serving you. It is time for a new one. Realizing that you want a different approach is the first step in creating a new path.

Desire to Change

> "Do it for me. I am trusting you to give me the body and experience that I want. I do not want any responsibility for having to do this. Make it easy. Make it fun. Make me see results. Success is to my credit, and failure, well, that is on you and whatever advice you gave me."

This is how some people approach personal trainers and health coaches. In fact, this is an outlook that one can have in various areas of life: a career, a relationship, or fitness. The absurdity is easier to see when it relates to the body. No one else is responsible for your success. Others can offer words of encouragement or the tools that worked for them. But you, only you, can make changes both mentally and physically. Only you can feel out what works. Only you can decide this is what you want! The desire and the commitment must come from within.

If you ever find yourself thinking those counterproductive thoughts or saying those words, try to recognize the absurdity in that moment. Real progress cannot be made until you take responsibility, until you take ownership of yourself.

A New Training Program

What does a conditioned mindset look like, think like, and how can you train yours? Let's consider a thought that represents the epitome of living all in—with a mindset that will seek out and create a life of fitness and physical well-being. Notice how you react to it.

"I enjoy moving my body and feeling vitality."

How did that feel to hear? Did you scoff? Roll your eyes? Did you quickly jump to list reasons why this is not true for you? Or maybe it felt light and refreshing. Maybe you said, "Yes, that's exactly how I want (keyword want) to feel." Better yet, were you thinking, "Well, of course! That's only natural." These responses represent some of the different ways we can approach fitness. These thoughts live in minds that have been trained in different ways. Can you guess which represents someone who enjoys working out? How about someone who lacks motivation? Can you envision people who embody each of these perspectives?

For some, seeing people that approach fitness in an enthusiastic way induces feelings of jealousy or disgust. Guess what? If that is your emotional response, it is a clear indicator that your mindset is in bad shape and likely injured. You are practicing and training in a way that is detrimental to your goals. You need to heal. You need to recover and start in a new direction. Start a new training program.

A training program is meant to get you in shape and invigorate new growth. The goal is improvement. But understand something—mental training is not only happening when action is taken. It also did not just begin. You train your mind every moment of every day. You can decondition or condition it. The difference is whether your mindset is taking you in the direction of what you want. The key is alignment. While this could be the moment a new seed is planted, there may already be firmly rooted weeds. The intention is not to de-weed the entire garden, but rather to create the space for a new flower to grow. Let's move forward to create the space to distinguish what it is we intend to grow.

Default Motivators

When we first embark upon training our mind in a new direction, three default motivators typically emerge. These concepts are often so embedded in our approach toward our bodies and fitness that many times people assume they are the only way. In fact, they are frequently considered to be interchangeable with a life of well-being. They may be fragments of the end result, but do not come close to capturing the foundation and core of living all in. Sure, they can be incorporated at a later point, but these default motivators can actually be holding you back. It is important that the seed we are planting is distinguished from these and given space to grow on its own. The three concepts are competition, looks, and health.

Competition

We grow up with an approach toward physical activity that is often centered around competition and comparison. This approach becomes a large factor in what motivates us, but is a double-edged sword.

Sports can provide entertainment and enjoyment. We are, however, as a society sports-obsessed.

Throughout adolescence, many have been unknowingly taught that fitness is synonymous with competition. Think back to when you were a child in school. The primary way in which we were encouraged to get in shape and be active was through athletic organizations. Athlete vs. athlete. Team vs. team. Even many of the physically active games we played at recess and during gym teach this approach. Through continual exposure to the games as the primary motivation for activity, we learn to associate fitness with comparison and competition. After all, it is the team with the most capable athletes that wins. Those who achieve victory, we assume, have the most fun.

This is not to say that we should completely remove competition or to suggest that everyone in a game be proclaimed a winner. There are some wonderful lessons that can be learned through athletics and team dynamics. However, it should not be at the core of our approach toward fitness. Incorporating competition into our concept of well-being and vitality can do more harm than good. A healthy foundation is built upon an internal relationship and self-worth, not upon beating others down.

Competition seeks to derive value through being better than another. Only by cutting someone down can we be elevated. There will be a time when someone performs better than you. Extracting your worth from being superior to another puts you in a vulnerable position to have your worth taken away.

Sometimes this can be seen among retired professional athletes. They constructed their sense of self-worth and idea of physical well-being on competition. Then, after they are out of the game, and not performing at such high levels, some lose motivation to stay in shape. Many times they feel as though they lost themselves. Their identity was built upon the hallowed ground of comparison.

For some, competition works temporarily. Failure, to another, can drive one to push harder. Yet there is no meaning there, and eventually they will fail. Eventually they will lose and not be able to get back up with the same mental motivation as before. How shallow, how meaningless, to only derive validation from others' losses? What's interesting is that some of the best athletes don't compete with others. Sure, to the spectator they do, but it isn't the predominant thought in the athlete's mind. They respect their so-called competitors.

The real focus, the real goal, is improving themselves. To get in their "zone," where they are in touch with their bodies. Where their mind reinforces their capabilities and calls their bodies to perform in miraculous ways.

What they are capable of is focus. Not on doubt or what others think. This is when they are the most successful. Shouldn't this be the main lesson we teach through athletics? Getting in touch with our bodies and our vitality in such a powerful way. Not to compete or be better than others, but to have the mind of the athlete. To be athletic doesn't mean one has to be comparing. Take the best athlete out of the ring, out of the stadium, out of the game, and their mind is still athletic. It is vigorous. It is agile. It is focused. It is conditioned.

When training your mindset to live a healthy and active lifestyle, competition won't get you far. Why? Competition is a harsh approach, and can lead down counterproductive paths. First, the fear of failure prevents us from trying. Second, competition derives a sense of value based upon comparing ourselves to others. We therefore essentially set ourselves up for a superficial, and sometimes abusive, relationship with our own bodies.

Most people who struggle with living an active lifestyle are deterred by the prevalence of physical competition in our culture. A majority of the ways we have been taught to be active consist of competitive games. Why take part if you are not confident in your physical capabilities? You would be setting yourself up for failure and embarrassment. Through your failure, your value is stripped away and given to another. After all, the winner gains, and the loser loses.

However, there are activities and options for working out that do not directly involve competition. Nevertheless, if you perceive only the comparative nature of physical activities, you will fear that everyone is judging you even if the activity is not obviously competitive. You may go to a yoga class, but feel concerned about others' perceptions. Or you decide to go to a gym, only to be scared of what others will think of the weight you are lifting, or how you look when you're doing it. How will others judge your capabilities, your body's performance? It's hard for a gentle soul to find physical activity enjoyable in a social setting when this is the predominant perspective—when it is seen as entering into the rink of competition.

Perspective is relative. Not everyone perceives the same way that you do. Even if in your mind you are sure of it. Remember that you want to change. This is your life. This is your body. You do not have to compete. Do not let the thoughts of another impact how you live your life and enjoy your physical experience. You can walk a different path. There is another way.

Why don't we teach fitness centered around the self? Why don't we focus on the idea of vitality? What happened to the youthful disposition toward play? Running, jumping, moving, just for fun. Have we lost touch with this? Why? Was it because we shifted our value and attention onto competition and less on the simple and pure appreciation of movement, of life?

Looks

Immediately upon hearing the words *looks* and *fitness* a slew of preconceived notions and ideas come rushing to mind. What society perceives to be attractive. What you think is attractive, and how your body fits in relation to that image. Frustration emerges if you are not where you want to be. Fear of losing it emerges if you are. Perhaps thoughts of aging arise, or annoyances at seemingly superficial and egotistically driven actions. Looks are an unabashed default motivator.

The default motivator of our physical appearance can carry us through our youth as a reason to engage in a healthy and active lifestyle. We desire our bodies to look a certain way. Most of the time, it is in order to appeal to others and therefore feel good about ourselves. The focus is on the result, and the reason for taking action is literally superficial. The purpose does not even graze the concept of feeling vitality. Sure, one may experience more energy and feel invigorated after taking the action, but that is not the primary impetus.

As you move through time, this motivator can fade. Other obligations conflict with a superficial view of fitness. After all who can justify spending time on their looks over quality family time, or a promotion at work? Our bodies continue to change. The appearance of your body now is not the same appearance you had as a child. Sure, it is the same body, but the way it looks has altered dramatically. So why is this ever fluid, ever evolving, aspect of our image a foundational motivator? How could this motivator possibly endure and sustain us throughout life with the same fire and intensity that it does in our youth? The intensity fades because the meaning is lost.

Oftentimes, the way we perceive our body is based upon the evaluations of things that are outside of us. What society, our friends, family, and significant others deem to be attractive shape how we approach fitness. It determines what exercises we do, how many repetitions, and the frequency. Sometimes this can directly work against us. Take, for instance, a woman who has somewhat weak bones. She should be doing resistance and weight-bearing exercises to strengthen them. However, she mistakenly fears getting "bulky," so she doesn't. She is more concerned with being attractive than listening to what her body needs, and therefore makes a series of uneducated assumptions. Letting this default motivator guide our actions takes the attention away from finding a movement that we enjoy, connecting to our vitality, and listening to our body. Instead, it is about what will appeal to others. What physical results will make them, supposedly, pleased. Goals are then constructed around what we imagine others think.

How backwards is that? How can the opinion that others hold about your physical appearance control how you approach the internal relationship you have with yourself? The focus should not be on training your body to be pleasing to others.

On the contrary, what if it is not just about our looks? What if the actions were a way to practice feeling good and invigorated? What if it was a way to celebrate life? Appearance would be the by-product of those actions. Is it selfish to care about how you feel? Is it selfish to want to experience your vitality and enjoy the by-products? How can you possibly ever uplift others if you do not do it for yourself? You cannot give what you do not have. We need to get away from the notion that being selfish in this way is a bad thing.

Enjoying the image and appearance of your body is not a bad thing. In fact, it is encouraged so long as the primary focus is on you and your body. Not what others think. Initially this will likely be a challenging concept because of your current state of mind. Therefore, to start, it ought not be your focus. There needs to be distance between your concept of physical image and this new seed you are planting.

Health

Would it come as a surprise if someone told you that one day you will leave this physical body? That one day your body will die? No, it wouldn't shock you. Why, then, are some people so focused on exercising solely for their health?

Most people are convinced that their body will one day become crippled. They focus only on the past and future, not the present. Their mindset is governed by thoughts of what they used to be capable of and what they fear lies ahead. Aging, then, becomes the reason nothing can improve and makes suffering inevitable.

We should not be motivated to live a healthy lifestyle out of fear of death or illness. Living healthfully merely to prolong your lifespan or avoid an ailment is a perspective built upon fear. It is preventative. It views the present through the lens of impending doom.

Fear is a strong emotion. It can provoke you to act, and it can prevent action. However, fear is meant to be an intense yet fleeting experience—an experience that redirects you. As a constant motivator, fear becomes counterproductive. It induces stress and anxiety: a concoction for decreased wellness.

Sure, there is a plethora of research indicating that a healthy, active lifestyle increases longevity, bolsters quality of living, and strengthens the immune system. However, viewing fitness as a means to prevent your well-being from diminishing is not a very cheerful, inspiring, or enjoyable notion. It's not that the body is unchangeable or impervious; rather, it's that focusing on how age has or will cripple your health is a terrible approach to living.

Knowing and feeling that something is good for your body—and then taking action—is one thing. Taking action simply to prevent an undesired consequence is another. The focus is different. The experience is different.

Unless their mindset goes beyond mere prevention, people who try to change their lifestyle because of an ailment (one that either they or a loved one experienced) usually give up. Their mindset must shift so that the change itself is wanted. That is the key. Without that change, struggle and defeat will follow.

Do not work out just for your health. You already are healthy. Did you hear that? At the core of your being, you are alive and vibrant. Is there air in your lungs? Blood in your veins? Of course there is! If not, you wouldn't be reading this book. You are predominantly healthy. You *have* health. You *are* health. You *are* life! Invigorating vitality is flowing through you, and if it wasn't, you would not be here. So, when you think about being physically active, look at it this way: Do not do it *for* your health. Do it to *feel* your health. There is a significant difference between these two approaches. Feeling your health leads to enjoyment. It leads to elevated experiences. Being physically active for your health is mundane, whereas doing it to feel your health is invigorating. It also brings your attention to the present and allows you to appreciate what you do have.

Regardless of the way your body looks, how much it weighs, or its physical capabilities, you can use it to tap into this feeling of vitality. Just step back for a minute and consider all the things your body does without your involvement. Consider all the things it does right.

There are a myriad of systems working in harmony within the body. The body is a miraculous feat of engineering that scientists are still grappling to understand. But most people are completely unaware, and therefore ungrateful, for the wellness they do have. Even when you are fighting a cold, your body is still healthy. It is still operating from a state of health without you recognizing it.

The body provides you with the opportunity to experience this world. It supports you. It has never failed you, and you have never failed it. Even if it gets sick, and even when it dies, it does not fail you. It is here to temporarily serve you. It will adapt and adjust. Remind yourself of the gifts that it gives you every day and at every moment.

When we say *feel health*, what we are really saying is to feel life—the miraculous, divine flow. To connect with your natural vitality. Imagine going for a walk because your doctor told you to. Now imagine going for a walk because it is a celebration of your existence in this body. The activity is the same, but the focus makes all the difference.

Feeling Good

Envision a triangle in which each point contains one of these concepts: competition, looks, and health. These motivators comprise the outlook that most people hold regarding well-being and fitness.

They are superficial ideas falling short of the true, deeper meaning and keep us focused in a way that is backwards. We are trained to force action first, with a default motivator as the reason. We are instructed to focus on the finish line as the reason for the experience.

These peripheral ideas surround what lies in the center. What is the reason we want to compete? What is the reason we want to look attractive? Why do we want to feel healthy? The underlying answer to all of these questions is that we want to feel good. We are seeking movement in a positive direction, either to obtain a state of being, or further the experience of it.

Are you starting to get a glimpse of what this new seed will blossom into? Understanding the distinctions and shortcomings of previous attempts, can you begin to see what was missing? Reorienting our mindsets will shift the approach from default motivation, to enthusiastic inspiration. That change will produce a different experience. It is not about anyone or anything other than you. It is your relationship with yourself, and in turn with the body you inhabit.

Experience and realize your vitality from a place of appreciation for this life and the body taking you along for the ride. With this as your foundation, the rest will naturally fall into place, such as your level of enjoyment, health, capabilities, and physical appearance. All of those manifestations branch out easily and joyfully from this place; not the other way around. When your perspective is focused more in the opposite direction, you will feel the struggle and meaninglessness of your efforts.

Bo's Story

Growing up, I was always involved in youth sports programs. I wasn't the fastest or the best athlete; nevertheless, I enjoyed playing. However, upon entering high school, competition was taken to new levels. Coaches expected more. More practices and better performances. Training at 6 a.m. and weight lifting after school. I especially remember despising working out. While it got results, it was also grueling, boring, and completely forced. As I graduated high school, my perspective on living a healthy and active lifestyle was flawed. But how could this be given that I was going to college to be a health and physical education teacher?

During my college years, I would work out with roommates. Competition was no longer the driving force, so what was? My ego. Yes, I knew exercise would keep me healthy, but it also made me look good. It wasn't until after I graduated that my perspective shifted.

One day, Daniella invited me to go for a run with her. Something she had started doing, and began casually expressing her enjoyment for. But, me running? Was I crazy? I would only lift weights occasionally. But what the heck, I would give it a shot. She seemed to enjoy it.

I approached my first runs as if I needed to push and make myself run faster and longer. It was, after all, my competitive training coming through. All the while Daniella, looking somehow refreshed by the activity, kept telling me to do it with ease. Have fun with it. It is natural for the body. Keep your feet light and just appreciate that we have access to such a beautiful place to run. What she was saying and how she was feeling about the process resonated with me.

As I went back to that same park, I was inspired to run longer and faster. I started eating healthier, working out regularly, and learning more about the body. The motivation wasn't to compete or look good. Rather, I just wanted to feel good and fitness became a way for me to connect with that and remind myself how awesome life really is. I didn't set out to change my mindset. I set out to have fun. And, ironically enough, I became the person I had been trying to inspire my students to be.

Two

Giving Up the Struggle

Breaking the Habit

We come to a place where the desire for change is evident. There is an idea of what we are after and understand it is both the journey and destination. So, how to change?

The traditional approach says to correct our habits. This is somewhat helpful and can impose a shift in the actions we take, hoping that the inspiration will eventually follow. There was a story of a man who could not seem to wake up for work on time. He forcefully broke the habit of oversleeping by parking behind his wife's car. Since she had to leave before him, he was forced to wake up and move his car before she left. He hated every moment of it, was miserable company, but did it for the result he wanted.

This approach can work for some as a way to force action, or for a short period of time. However, it is not actually breaking the habit. It is only trying to combat it, or overpower it, which often causes the habit to become more deeply entrenched. What a terrible approach to life! Life is precious. To dredge through it, forcing yourself to do things that you hate is not very meaningful or enjoyable. The problem with trying to change only our physical habits, without addressing our mindset, is that we are not shifting how we experience the situation or the activity. There is still internal resistance to the very things we want, and it can be felt as hopelessness, frustration, or resentment. As much as we attempt to coerce our habits to change, we strongly try to find ways to justify or excuse ourselves from that commitment. We need to align our mindset with how we wish to experience life. The action will grow from that fertile soil.

When it comes to fitness, we often see people forcing action when their mental and emotional state are not aligned. They try to make themselves work out or diet because they desire certain results. Yet, they hate every second of it. All the while, they despise and blame their bodies for making them have to go through it. This causes an unhealthy relationship between the self (body and mind). There is this notion that action trumps everything. That we need to aggressively make our bodies be and behave in a way we desire them to.

Punishment Perspective

When exercise is viewed or treated as a way to aggressively and forcefully change the body, there is an internal disconnect. The mind is at war with the body. The relationship between the two is not connected with a mutually beneficial interest in thriving. There is disconnect, and the mind seeks to punish the body into submission.

Sound a little harsh? That's because it is. Consider anytime action is taken because the body is viewed as inadequate. Because it disgusts or frustrates its owner. Anytime action is taken from that place of being insufficient or "wrong," there is a strong chance that the body is being perceived as inappropriate. Most of the time this is weight related, but can span to a variety of abilities or characteristics. This is something to be aware of as we focus on the relationship we have with ourselves.

With this approach, the body's natural indicators are suppressed and ignored. Its messages are disregarded, as if you were wronged by its weight or apparent lack of capabilities. This is when people are more likely to be injured, because they ignore the body's signals, and ultimately isn't that what a punishment is meant to do? To injure the other in the relationship so they are submissive. In this case, the other is the body. This is not to say that you will never get injured as you move through life. However, it is less likely if you are in tune with your body. You will learn to better distinguish between the tension or ache of a good workout, and the pain of injury. The timing of when to call your body to new performance heights, and when to ease into it can only be discovered by listening to the body.

There is this concept of "no pains, no gains," but you are not going to keep doing something that is painful. And if you are consistently in pain, you probably won't be able to. Pushing yourself to the next level can be a little uncomfortable, which is why it is considered out of your comfort zone. But painful? No. Painful means injury. It means carelessness. There is a distinction to be made between the punishment perspective and how someone with an all in mindset approaches progress.

When we "push ourselves," there is a difference in motivation. Pushing yourself based on the punishment perspective is beating yourself up. Driving yourself based on enjoyment and the belief that you can do more, that you desire to do more, is calling your body toward elevation. The mind is conditioned. Can you feel the difference between these two approaches? The punishment perspective forces the body to move us forward by pushing it from behind. On the other hand, calling your body toward action puts the mind ahead and asks the body to join in the experience.

Oftentimes exercise-fad or bandwagon individuals struggle with this distinction. They are only motivated by lack. Only when they think something is terribly wrong will they take action. Yet, being dependent upon struggle and the thrill of the chase doesn't teach someone how to maintain. It doesn't allow for continuous engagement. Once obtained, the movement is boring, unenjoyable, or not of primary importance.

Think of how many rally calls and plans are built around the fight to get in shape and be healthy. They are fueled by negativity. The reason so many people lack motivation to maintain is that they don't know what type of fuel to use when they aren't fighting anymore. They don't have the mindset to support success. They are trained to use negativity, but have not yet grasped the infinite energy of positivity and enthusiasm. They have not learned how to shift gears and continue the journey. This is why we must train our minds as well as our bodies.

But what about gently correcting or adjusting? If we don't like the situation or condition of our body, can't we take action to change it? The difference is the place from which the action is taken and the mind's role in creating it. The difference is either full alignment or discord.

Making Peace

Who can you blame for you? For how you live. For what you know. For how you view yourself. Who can you blame? Well, of course I can blame my parents and family for not knowing any better and withholding opportunities. I can blame my friends for perpetuating the cycle and exposing me to their failures. I can blame my genes and my circumstances. Heck, I can even blame my job. I can blame anything and anyone for getting me to the point where I am now. Great! I completely evaded responsibility. So, now what?

You are at the intersection of change. But in order to pivot, in order to go in a new direction, which may consist of gradual turns, there is one thing that needs to happen—you must make peace with the past.

What does that mean? Does it mean rehashing everything? Or finding excuses and places to put blame? Or beating yourself up about how you didn't do this sooner? No, contrary to what many people think of making peace with the past, the way we use the phrase actually is intended to have little emphasis on the word *past* and more on the word *peace*.

You must decide that you want something different. And then you must move in the direction of what you want. But you cannot do that if you don't believe you have any control over you. You cannot do that if you let people, experiences, and circumstances from your past take away your power now. In this moment, they are no longer responsible for you. What your parents taught you about health and fitness is no longer responsible for how you move forward. The experiences of embarrassment or frustration are no longer responsible for you not trying.

Where you are now. How you feel now is not anyone or anything's fault. Reclaim your power to choose how you want to live. You are free to choose a different experience. You are free to move in a new direction.

Making peace with the past is really not about the past. It is about this moment and being not just responsible for yourself, but being in your power—being empowered. The two words actually go hand in hand. Being response-able means determining how you choose to respond both internally and externally. What you choose to think, say, and feel about the topic of fitness and health is deliberate. You are response-able, not disabled. You are not disabled by the past, by what others think, or by what others believe you are capable of. You are not dis-abled by anything. You are responsible for yourself. And when you are in the moment able to intentionally respond, you are in your power. Because it is then that you can create the experience, the perspective, the mentality that breeds success.

Three

All In

Response-ability can only be implemented in the present moment. Deciding to move in a new direction, mentally and physically, can only be initiated now.

The idea of just doing something is great, if you're all in. All in refers to wanting what you're doing, when you're doing it. It involves being mentally, physically, and emotionally aligned. It is bringing all of you to the present situation. These three aspects support and guide the action. You are completely committed, fully integrated. This doesn't mean you're rigidly fixated on only one goal or way of moving forward. In fact, many times being all in requires the ability to adjust, flexibility in order to shift gears, and the presence of mind to sense or know when to do so.

People think being fully committed means being determined and driven to make a result happen, no matter what. However, most people looking to get in shape have a deconditioned mind that turns that approach into punishing their body. They push and ignore their body while self-defeating thoughts consume or tangle the mind. For example, "This isn't working. I'm not fit enough. I'm too old for this." Or perhaps they are focused on all the things they would rather be doing.

Taking action when the mind is preoccupied with those types of thoughts is only partial commitment. The body is taking the action, but the mind doesn't support it. In fact, the mind hinders the body and prevents a positive experience. This paves the way for future situations to yield the same negative outlook. Is it any wonder why a mind in that state would perceive the situation as unpleasant?

Someone who enjoys a healthy, active lifestyle has a conditioned mindset and practices being all in.

Their joy, their seeming effortlessness, is the indicator. Initially one with a deconditioned mind would find being all in challenging. The soil of their mind is poisoned with old thoughts about fitness and the body. These need to be gradually replaced with new, fertile beliefs and ideas. That process will shift the approach and provide the foundational support to start moving in a new direction.

What Is Normal?

Normal is typically dictated by what the average number of people you are surrounded by experience. But what if dysfunction is the norm? Do you want to be mediocre in your dysfunction? Or do you want to thrive in the function of your natural state?

What is normal? What is the body's natural state? Those questions induce blanket generalizations and a mesh of assumptions based upon the experiences of others and your past. However, your body and the way you experience it is uniquely yours. As discussed, you are response-able for yourself. No one else can inhabit your body or decide that you feel a particular way in it. You cannot transfer your health or feeling of vitality to another who is lacking it, just as you cannot force another to feel good in their own skin. The experience is uniquely individual. So let's take others out of the equation and clarify that question.

What do you consider to be your body's natural state? Is that state your normal experience? Is it natural for you to be predominately well or sick? Is it normal for you to feel vibrant and energized? Is it normal for you to feel lethargic? Sure, there may be fluctuations, but what is your experience most of the time? Take a second to ponder those questions.

Whatever someone considers to be normal represents their typical way of experiencing life and their body. It also reflects their expectations, whether they have high or low standards. For a smoker who has frequent coughing fits, coughing becomes their normal. They will not seek to change if they accept it as ordinary. With that acceptance, their standards are lowered. Only when an experience is outside of the norm, or below that threshold, do most people recognize the need for adjustments. Some people dread working out and believe it is normal to feel that way. Some think it is normal to feel tired after eating. Others expect to feel energized. With low baseline standards, the experience must be deprived before the desire for adjustments is acknowledged. Or, the standards must be questioned and the expectations raised.

If you believe your body's natural state is ill or fragile, you are going to treat it as such, vigilantly standing watch for something to go wrong. You will not see what is going right and then appreciate what you have, because your gaze will be fixed on impending doom.

Nearly everyone has encountered someone who does not seem capable of being well. One thing after another is wrong with them, as though they need some ailment to complain about or they wouldn't have anything to talk about. Even a paper cut becomes life altering to this personality. They see their natural state as sick or injured. They believe themselves to be victims of their weak bodies. They do not know another way of existing and, one could speculate, do not want another way because their identity is so closely tied to things going wrong. For people like this, ailment is their standard.

Those with an all in mindset believe that their natural and predominate state is well. They emanate and seek out that wellness. There is also an understanding that the body is made to move. They do not dread physical activity, because to them it is natural. What is natural, feels good.

Naturally Well

The body's natural state is well. It is healthy, energized, and vibrant. Furthermore, you should expect to feel good in it. Any form of injury or sickness is an oddity, a slight deviation from its natural well-being. Sure, there may be times when this is challenged and medical guidance is needed. The main difference is that even during challenging times, someone living all in will be able to recognize and appreciate the wellness that still exists within the body. Even if it is just a glimmer. They seek a path that supports the body in healing. Perhaps there is a little frustration, but that does not consume them. Their energy is directed toward solutions and on improving their experience, rather than complaining about it. They move forward, soothing the mindset and body so their attention can remain on celebrating life and feeling good. As mentioned previously, you are health. It is something to live, not obtain. It is something to experience, a state of being.

Simply recognizing that it is normal and natural to feel healthy and good reestablishes your base standard, or set point. It raises your expectations, and along with raised expectations comes an increased sensitivity toward living in harmony with that wellness.

When you come to understand your body's natural state as well, you are more inclined to get in touch with it and listen to its natural indicators. When something is off, you'll feel out what it needs or seek assistance. An awkward movement doesn't have to become an injury because you tried to bulldoze through it for the sake of your looks or ego. You notice the movement feels odd, adjust, and likely avoid the problem all together.

You will be more inclined to notice a tight muscle and seek to release it. Or notice you're thirsty for more water as your immune system is ramped up. Why? Because knowing the body is naturally well, it seeks equilibrium and realignment.

You partner with your body in experiencing this life. From there, you look for ways to not only connect with vitality, but exude it. Emanate it with actions and decisions. This is the solid foundation, the fertile soil in which vibrant, joyful, physical actions grow. It is the difference between exercising because you have to and dancing because you want to.

Made to Move

As a society, we have come to a point where many people are not required to move. Our jobs and entertainment are largely static. Obtaining food and enjoying comforts does not require a significant exertion of energy. After all, most aren't tilling fields for produce, hulling lumber to make a home, or hunting for dinner. The thing is, with all this progress many have forgotten what their bodies were designed to do—move!

We are not planted like flowers and trees. Sitting for days on end is not normal and typically not natural—moving is. Our bodies were made to be in motion. Recognizing this simple fact will begin to reframe your choices. You will be more inclined to get up and take action if you believe it is natural. Just as the body adapts based on the training you put it through, it will become deconditioned if ignored. Moving invigorates the body. Feeling energized is the expectation. Start practicing what is natural—get moving!

Focus on Abilities

If you were walking into a job interview, would you focus on what you couldn't do in order to land the position? Would you rattle off every skill you don't have and why you're determined not to try and obtain them? Or discuss every obstacle in your way? No, you would focus on the skills you do have and how they could translate. If you were on a first date, would you spew out every criticism you ever received? Or emphasize why others' heartbreaks are holding you back from love? Hopefully not! While these examples seem ridiculous, that is the whole point. Yet some people apply this approach toward their bodies.

The focus is on what they can't do, instead of what they can do. This emphasizes limitations and excuses. It attempts to justify all the reasons that they can't be healthy, active, and consistently in touch with their vitality. There has to be a shift in focus toward what is possible, what is achievable, and what you are capable of doing. Maybe your condition right now prevents you from lifting weights, but you are able to go for a walk. Perhaps you are capable of swimming. Maybe lack of movement is making your condition worse instead of better. You have to look for ways to work within your means, right here and now. Recognize your current situation. However, keep your gaze focused on improvement. There are so many options, but if you are fixated on the problem, you won't let in the solution.

Most people are not aware of how much wellness they are actually living. The phrase "taking it for granted" falls short as it assumes a high level of expectation. There should be a high level of expectation regarding wellness. However, going unnoticed it is unable to develop into something that can be appreciated, and fully enjoyed. Exercise and train the mind by the power of your focus. What you give your attention to is what the mind is trained toward. This can be seen in how one approaches their capabilities, internal dialogue, and how they view circumstances.

Say "Yes"!

Constantly saying "no" creates a mindset of deprivation. Perhaps it is the thought that exercise deprives you of time to relax. Or, if you are being more conscious about food choices, that you are deprived of tasty treats. That associates your new actions and decisions with lack. As we know by now, that is not the disposition of a some-one living all in. Reframing your choices presents a different way of perceiving, and therefore responding to a decision.

Shift the focus onto what you'll gain from taking the desired course of action. This will gradually retrain the decision-making process. The mind will be taught to identify and perceive the benefits beforehand. This creates an association between the action or behavioral choice and obtaining a desired state of being. When you change what the mind is fixated on, you alter your mind-set. The mind is then set to seek out actions and make decisions that align with how you desire to live. You are conditioning the mind to live in harmony with health and vitality.

When making a choice to go in a new direction, the emphasis needs to be on what is wanted. Start noticing and focusing on saying "yes." When you think about going for a jog, you're saying "yes" to feeling invigorated! You're saying "yes" to feeling your health! You're saying "yes" to feeling good! Instead of saying "no" to a cupcake, you could say "yes" to a bowl of fruit and to nourishing the body. Rather than denying yourself things, look for what you are giving to yourself.

Granted there are days when the best course of action for the body is to rest. Listen to that. Don't deny yourself a workout. Say "yes" to rejuvenation. It is only temporarily needed. Do you see the difference? This creates the all in approach. You are mentally, emotional, and physically committed to your choice. However, the decision always follows what aligns with a feeling of wellness.

It may be tempting for some to excuse themselves from following through by manipulating this approach.

Only you know the intentions behind your choices. There is not a blanket prescription for when to rest and when to take action. Strategies and techniques for transforming laziness and low energy levels will be discussed later in the book. For now, recognize the value in reframing your choices.

Self-talk

Why put yourself down? If someone tells you what they dislike about their body, do not feel socially obligated to list things you think are wrong with yours just to fit in. There may be a few trouble spots on your mind, but let gratitude redirect your focus. Limit how often and how much you talk about perceived problems. Don't give those unproductive thoughts air time. That simply spreads weeds and reinforces the old perspective of self-loathing and criticism. The objective is to foster a positive relationship with your body, your vitality, and encourage onward progress.

This may seem daunting because one can think so many counterproductive thoughts on a topic and have no idea how to control them, or change them for that matter. It can seem near impossible if that approach has been practiced for a long period of time. We recommend a gentle method. Heal your thoughts. Going from dreading to loving something is too far of an emotional stretch. But there needs to be improvement and growth in the desired direction. So instead of saying you hate something, heal your words to say something like:

"It's not so bad. I am going to be glad I did this. Doing this takes me down the path that I want. This is good for my body. This is natural."

Being aware of the things you tell yourself, and even others, about the topic is important to establishing a new mindset. Aside from changing your perspective on working out, it is important to be aware of what you are telling yourself about your body. Remember, your body is naturally well. You are health. You are vitality. Be grateful for your body, and this life.

Appreciating is the bridge. Find some part of your body that is working and be grateful for it. Focus on that one aspect and appreciate its vitality in this moment. Be grateful it is functioning and that you have been given it as a gift, as a way to experience this life and world. Regardless of any condition, can you feel gratitude for the life you were given?

Tip the Scale

Tip the scale. Not the weight scale. Tip the perspective scale. To clarify, this isn't weighted over a period of time, as people often think. Nor is it keeping a journal of how many times you felt in touch with your vitality. It is gauging where you are at any given moment, which requires presence and awareness. Where are you putting your weight? Are you throwing it towards what you want, or the lack thereof? Every second, are your actions and thoughts supporting the mentality you want? Sure, while you are working behind a desk it can be hard to take aligned action, but what about the food you're putting in your body? What about the ideas you're thinking in regards to your body and movement? Those are things that get thrown on this scale, too. Tip the balance in your favor.

What you repeatedly tell yourself becomes what you believe. When deliberately changing the way you approach fitness, you have to start telling yourself new things. There has to be a new story surrounding the action taken. There has to be new thoughts that support the mindset you are creating. Athletes do this all the time, but to a greater degree because they have more momentum on the subject. They pump themselves up! They are deliberate about creating an atmosphere for themselves and are selective about the thoughts they tell themselves. They repeatedly affirm their capabilities—purposefully get excited and energized. It is the same concept, but at a slower pace. Remember, we are training the mind, and once it has established a certain level of fitness we can amp it up.

The Most Important Relationship

Knowing your natural state, the way the body is perceived and therefore engaged, changes. It becomes a wonderful vessel through which life is experienced and exuded. Invigorated by its movements. Inspired by its ability to feel the sensations of living. A harmonious relationship develops, and just like any relationship a commitment and decision to nurture it is necessary.

For some looking to find rhythm and balance in both their approach and actions, the concept of a designated time to cheat may be tempting. However, who is being cheated—yourself? Your body? Relationships are built upon trust and commitment. The practice of cheating negates that foundation. That is not an aligned mindset. That is not living all in.

To cheat implies that there is a release of tension or an urge that built up. An unpleasant escalation is an indicator of internal resistance. Rather than being all in, there is discord. Seeking absolution means that you are not really enjoying the new path and staying committed to yourself. However, this is the way some people have come to understand balance.

That is not balance. Forbidding all supposed vices is not balanced, either. Savoring treats on occasion is okay and so is resting. A gymnast doesn't walk three-fourths the way down a beam and then jump off because she cannot keep her balance anymore. She has to be able to keep walking, and even if sometimes there is a little wobble she still has strong footing. Maybe sometimes she feels as if she is going to fall off all together, but she refocuses, gets centered, and keeps going—moving forward. That's what it means to live in balance.

Only after a self-commitment has been made and a deep desire to live one's health is ignited can this natural balance evolve. Becoming more sensitive to maneuvers that throw you off center, and learning to adjust, are skills that develop with practice.

Gradually a shift takes place. You will seek food choices that nourish and invigorate. Rather than focusing primarily on how something tastes on the tongue, you'll become increasingly aware of how it impacts you. How it feels. It will no longer feel good to overindulge in nutrient-lacking foods. It will no longer feel good to be lethargic. The temporary comfort found in those old habits are nothing compared to the joy of liveliness. Lifestyle choices become aligned with your natural state. Drab physical activities will become colorful and vibrant. Cravings for nutrient-rich foods and exercise emerge. Listening and following natural inclinations foster from this place of knowing wellness. As the level of enjoyment increases, so does the appreciation for it. Rather than training to become something, you are it. The actions are natural extensions, examples, that align with you.

As you progress, those around you will see you as a person with good habits. But these are not mindless, repetitive actions. They are deliberate. They are fun and enjoyable. They are extensions of a way of living—all in.

This is, however, a process. Is it possible that you will instantaneously change? Yes, it is possible. After all, any momentary experience occurs in an instant. Either way, you have to continue to nurture this new mindset and redirect actions and thoughts that would otherwise hinder its growth. If you know yourself at the core of your being, as wellness, then your thoughts, actions, and body will rise to meet your expectations.

Four

EVOLVING GOALS

Creating the Way

Goals are not a bad thing. However, they should not be the entire focus. After all, they usually don't reflect a consistent way of living. Most people create goals that center around crash diet and exercise plans. Within one week they want to lose five pounds, or within one month they want to get lean and build muscle. Even if they do achieve a temporary goal, they quickly fall back into their past lifestyles. These are rollercoaster goals. They aim high and fall short. Even if they hit their target, they are not sustained and the journey is tense and forced.

We are now at a place where we are taking our mental training and living it—implementing it into aligned action. One could say the goal is to live all in and get in touch with their vitality, but that is not what a goal should be. That is how you wish to live. A way of being. A goal should be derived from this, not the other way around. Goals are temporary. They should be helpful ways of keeping us on the path. Keeping the journey fun, fresh, and exciting. However, that is not the way we are used to conceiving and generating them.

For some the word *goal* conjures the image of an egotistical, dominating personality. For example, the person determined to rise the ranks at work or the person driven to achieve physical fitness for the sake of their ego. A hyper-specific way of shaping life that involves action plans, deadlines, and stress. What you determined were your goals yesterday and what you thought was the best way of achieving them, rigidly dictates how you act in the future. This is without any regard for adaptability and mental training.

But what about when challenges arise? Let's take for example a man who sets a goal to go for a run three times a week and wants to build up to a specific distance. He starts off doing well. He will run outside when possible, and indoor on his gym's treadmill when it is not. But then a winter storm rolls in. A blizzard covers his town and makes it impossible to navigate his way to the gym. Running is not an option this week. What does he do? He technically failed his goal. Will he beat himself up or feel agitated with his inability to do what he wants? Well, if his goal is intentionally pulled from his broader way of being, then circumstances will not deter him. He will persevere and find another means of expressing it. Knowing that his overall focus is on a way of living, he shrugs off the snow and makes the most of the situation. Instead he does some yoga and indoor body weight exercises.

Or what about the person who fought hard to shed weight and get toned only to lose motivation once it was achieved. She started slipping and ended up back where she began. Her goal was specific and obtainable, but not continual. It lacked a framework and mentality to support ongoing success.

Goals are merely a reflection, an expression, of your way of life. They are not the entire thing. They do not encompass your existence. Rather they are fun ways of identifying and then creating what you want. They are physical expressions of how to live your desired state.

For someone living all in, there is no such thing as a diet. There is no such thing as a crash exercise plan. Sure there are fluctuations, but there is consistency and oftentimes adaptability. New goals, or better stated, new adventures emerge as expressions of the desire to live feeling vitality. The goals are not required to continue moving forward because the framework of leading a healthy active lifestyle has already been established. New goals are simply an extension of a lifestyle and commitment to feeling good.

Guidelines for Creating Fitness Goals

1) *Focus on the feelings*. Goals should be a way to enrich and add excitement to the journey. Being in touch with your vitality is a way of being. What emotions does living in that way conjure within you? Consider those feelings. Write them down. State them out loud. Let those emotions marinate and become your desired way of being. You want this! Any goal should align with your overarching theme. Contemplating the desired feelings first sets your focus, sets your intention, on what really matters. This is an essential practice because it

reminds us that the way of being, is more important than the specifics. It allows for flexibility and continuity in approach. It provides us with a canvas on which to create. This is important to establish, especially when we are building a new perspective.

2) *Forget about the stats and focus on the movement.* Pay attention to the performance measuring up to your how. Most people are numbers obsessed, specifically with weight. As much as weight may be a primary motivating factor and source of great frustration, we urge you to put it aside when choosing goals. Focus on movement-based activities. For example, make your goal being able to complete a dance routine, a pull up, run the trail at a local park, or hold a yoga pose. Yes, it should be challenging to you. Yes, it should be something that you think is interesting. It should be something that when you witness another performing it, you are impressed. The movement represents the remarkability of the human body. Then, assess where you are and do your research. Look at what needs to be improved in your body and in your lifestyle in order to achieve your goal. This may also involve partnering with a professional for customized guidance. Embarking upon training

to complete the movement, you will find yourself engaging more parts of the body and using a more holistic approach. Someone who wants to do a yoga pose may find her arm strength increasing and posture improving. Perhaps she also identified and corrected muscle imbalances that prevented a full range of motion. Create goals that center around the awe-inspiring movements of the body, not merely a superficial number. Keep them fun and keep them fresh.

3) *Gauging an action plan*. Creating timelines and accountability check-ins may be helpful for some. If that assists you as a way of focusing, go for it! However, be honest. Will creating timelines shift your attention away from the broader way of being and introduce a punishment perspective? Will you become overly fixated on a result and not on training your mindset and living all in? You have to know yourself and feel out what style works best for you. A general rule of thumb is that if it feels exciting to contemplate a more specific plan, then it is right for where you are right now. Should a feeling of tension, unease, or frustration emerge, then for now stick to a general approach. The discomfort is an indicator

that your perspective is pointed in the direction of being insufficient. Building upon that will only cause resentment. Remember, goals are just extensions of how you wish to live. If they are pulled in this way, they light the inspired way of living already within you. Creating timelines and action plans are focusing tools. Don't focus on something that doesn't feel right to you.

Keep in mind that the path doesn't always take the course we thought it would. This can be applicable to any area of life. For example, when we first started writing this book, there was a general sense of when we wanted it completed. However, the state in which it was written and quality of content was more important than a due date. As we extended past the broad deadline, we realized that new ideas were emerging as a result of life experiences. If we rushed the process without regard for how it was unfolding, we would have missed out on core ideas.

Here is a fitness example. While practicing a dance routine, one may realize they have tight hamstrings and needs to increase flexibility. That wasn't taken into account during the initial timeline, but it needs to be if they want to continue.

The process cannot always be rushed, and mental training as well as getting physically in shape is a process. When starting something new, you are not an expert. That's what makes it fun! If you already had or were living your goal, it wouldn't be your goal! Don't get too wrapped up in deadlines. They are simply a way of making sure you're following through. Remember, how the journey feels is more important than the specifics.

Don't Overshare Your Goals

This completely goes against conventional wisdom. We have been taught to share our goals, especially the ones that seem to be the most challenging. To invite others' suggestions, advice, and criticism. We are taught that it will hold us accountable, provide a support network, and push us harder. If this works for you, great! However, chances are, if you are reading this book, it has not.

Most people who have struggled with the goal of fitness, weight loss, and maintaining an active lifestyle have not found this approach to work consistently and provide long-term results. Why would this be?

Remember that we are training the mind as well as the body. This is an incredibly personal experience. It is a relationship that you are in with yourself; no one else. Sharing your goals at this stage may not be helpful. It is typically encouraged for one of two reasons. First, to be accountable and push us harder. Second, to garner support and encouragement.

> "Sharing goals holds me accountable and drives me to achieve."

Sharing holds you accountable to the people you shared your goals with. It ups the ante by placing the fear of failure upon yourself. But you are not accountable to them. Too often we push ourselves in order to garner approval from others out of concern of what they think. When this happens, we introduce a punishment perspective, are less likely to get in touch with our bodies, and are less inclined to complete the action out of pure enjoyment for the movement.

> "Sharing with others will give me encouragement."

Sharing for encouragement typically takes you down one of two paths. The first, and more desired, is the initial rush of positivity and support derived from those around you. The thrill and excitement reaffirms the goal. That may temporarily feel motivating, but it is not permanent. Sharing to extract enthusiasm from others is not developing an internal relationship. It is deconditioning the mind. It is going in the wrong direction by teaching us to find motivation externally, not internally.

The second path that sharing for encouragement may lead to is being confronted with a doubter. This is someone who does not necessarily completely encourage or believe in you. When you begin the process of conditioning the mind, you are still building your momentum and creating a foundation. Opening yourself up to others' judgments, criticism, and doubts may set you back rather than propel you forward.

Starting out, you don't have the confidence or the momentum to stand in front of someone who doesn't completely believe in you, or truly care about you, and state your goals without your perspective faltering. Most of the time we are eager to share with those we are close to, or who we have known the longest. Unfortunately, those loved ones usually see through the lens of what you were or are, not what you will be. They know your past failures, and as much as they may love you, will sometimes see new goals through the lens of the past. We all know the look. When someone smiles and speaks words of support, but deep in their eyes you feel their lack of faith or judgment. Don't put yourself out there. Don't overexpose yourself as you begin to change the relationship that you have with yourself.

You have to practice this enough to be able to stand in front of someone who may judge or encourage you and not care about their reaction. You don't need to impress them. You don't need to prove anything, or even justify yourself. The interesting thing is that once you can firmly stand in this resolve, with momentum, you will want to share out of pure excitement and joy. It is not because anyone else needs to change. It is because you love this aspect of yourself so much that you will gladly share it.

Refrain from oversharing, especially in the beginning. It may be positioning you for a line of questioning and dialogue that diverts you from your path. When embarking upon a new goal, keep the first few steps private. It is a personal experience, and the roots are starting to take shape. It's all too easy to let publicized goals distract you back into old habits and approaches. Or redirect the focus away from the broader "how" that we discussed earlier.

You don't need to lie about what you're doing or where you're going. Simply refrain from sharing the internal value being placed upon those actions. For example, instead of broadcasting to coworkers your goals and plans to go for a jog after work, keep it to yourself. If someone asks where you are going, simply reply, "I am going for a jog." Whatever their response, keep yours simple and filled with excitement. Perhaps you could say, "It will feel good to get outside." Or, "After working, I just need to move my body." Leave it at that.

There is value in learning to find joy in the action and movement by yourself. We cannot depend on someone to always be there to pick us up and take us along for the ride. We have to learn it for ourselves. There can, however, be joy in sharing your journey with others. That being said, there are certain people to share goals with, if it feels right. And that is essential—it has to feel right.

Picky About Company

Be picky about who you share and surround yourself with. When a tennis player wants to get better at her game, who should she play with? Someone worse than her, an equal, or someone who is better at the game? If she wants to get better, she plays with someone better. The same holds true for improving your mindset.

Don't go for a hike or workout with just any partner. Be selective! You are inviting someone into the process of shaping your disposition. Don't go with someone who doubts their capabilities, complains, judges, or brings you and your efforts down. Go with someone who elevates, inspires, and encourages! Every time action is taken, the thoughts you have about it are shaping a new disposition. If you are going to invite a partner, choose someone with a more conditioned mind. Someone who has practiced their perspective to the point of ease, who sees you as capable of succeeding. This may be a personal trainer, a friend, or family member. The process should be fun. If it feels right, these are the people you can privately share your goals with.

Celebrate Others' Success

Have you ever seen someone in great shape and immediately felt jealous? Maybe you saw someone fit run past and in that moment disliked them. Perhaps a slew of judgmental thoughts crossed your mind. "They are too skinny, or too muscular. He must not have a life. She hasn't had kids yet, etc."

Instantaneously people compare and judge. Those bitter thoughts reflect self-loathing and the primary excuses you allow yourself. They illustrate your perspective and where the mindset needs to be retrained.

When condemnation, criticism, or negative emotions are directed at someone who exemplifies what you desire, the mind is being conditioned that it is a bad thing. In turn, you are training yourself to associate those discouraging feelings with the very things you want. This is reaffirming the perspective that you are seeking to displace. It poisons the soil of the mind and creates internal resistance.

Why would anyone condemn what they want? Well, it is not intentional. That is why awareness is needed. If we want taking action to be easier, if we want it to be fun, then we must celebrate others' achievements. Do you need to congratulate everyone you see at the gym, or personally like them? No, but the internal response should be positive. View their actions and capabilities as awe inspiring. Think to yourself, "Good for them! Wow, the body is capable of such beautiful movements. They have the passion toward working out that I want! They look focused and invigorated!"

On a tangible level, no one knows the work another puts in behind the scenes—their story, their goals, or progress. Perhaps the person you initially condemned for running past you started running a year ago after an illness. Or they worked their way up to that point after losing a lot of weight. Or maybe they are just naturally fit, in which case you would probably call them a few choice words. But why? Because for them it is effortless and enjoyable? Don't you see, they exemplify your desires? Their story shouldn't matter to you either way. The focus should be on the relationship you are in with yourself. If it helps to soften your disposition, recognize that you will never fully know another's story. It is not only counterproductive to your goals to criticize, but it is ill-informed. Ultimately seeing someone who has the physical and mental conditioning that you want is like crossing paths with a mentor. They can aid in identifying where you need training. If you allow it, they can also be a visual catalyst to garner more momentum toward the conditioning process. Be grateful for the experience!

Challenges

There may be times of polishing, but that polish only reveals the stone underneath. You have to be patient with the process. Otherwise, you will let go of a gem without realizing it.

As you grow this new seed, how will you respond if a weed appears? While developing a new approach, you will likely encounter challenges. They could take the shape of external circumstances, or internal thoughts.

These trials tend to be when people falter and give up. They allow a misstep to debilitate, believing their disappointment represents a sure sign of overall failure.

Remember those old habits are just repetitive thoughts—merely a simple idea or approach that was reiterated until it became your norm. The determining factor is how you respond. How do you treat yourself after a lapse in words, thoughts, or behaviors? How do you react? Much like a training exercise, challenges will demonstrate your weaknesses. They will also show your strengths. It is your response not only to the present moment but to yourself. Are you response-able? Are you able to deliberately remind yourself of the growing seed? Remind yourself of what it is you really want. Then, mentally shift and move in the direction of your desire.

The difference is that now you know better. Now you know that focusing on the weeds, grows the weeds. The harder you pull on them, the more rooted they become. Don't let a weed disable you.

Frustration

It is okay to feel frustrated after realizing you had a lapse in commitment. After all, you caught yourself living in contradiction to what you desire. Just don't stay frustrated. Transform the fiery emotion into fuel to help shift the direction in which you are pointed. Refrain from letting it push you further in the direction of what is unwanted. Don't let it control your focus. Upon beginning to change, and becoming aware of the importance of mindset training, people tend to get angry with themselves rather easily. They get frustrated when they "mess up."

They don't know how to quickly burn off their frustration and redirect their focus. Taking action without shifting your state, causes addiction to the catalyst of frustration. People then become dependent upon the burn-off fuel for motivation and sustenance. As you can see, this feeds the punishment perspective.

We are much too harsh on ourselves. How can you ever change if you don't recognize what it is that needs to change? You may not be mentally strong enough to completely pivot in a given moment, but you can make a series of gradual turns. With practice, those gradual turns will teach you to pivot. Eventually you will learn the movement. It will become easier, faster, and your starting point will shift so the pivot is to a lesser degree.

As crazy as it may sound, celebrate that awareness. You just recognized something that doesn't serve you and now have the power to change it. Surprisingly the emotion of frustration is closer to what you want than past feelings of hopelessness. Hopelessness assumes that what you desire is out of your control. Use that feeling of frustration to get you to a place of taking responsibility and recognizing your power—that you do have control and can work toward your own goals. Then, become present and able to determine how you want to move forward. Use frustration as a refocusing tool, and then let it go. Focus on your goal and the feeling you desire. The two go hand-in-hand as we have learned how a conditioned mindset allows us to achieve our goals.

Eye on the Prize

Keep your eye on the prize. Focus on what matters. Realize that getting stuck in the mentality of shortcoming and failures—of condemning yourself in ways big and small—is not going to produce the results you desire. Fixating on what went wrong is counterproductive. It wastes time and energy that could be used toward a solution.

Remember that every goal is an extension of your way of life. You must stay committed to that greater intention. That is the only way you will get back up and continue to grow the new perspective that will energize the new actions you need to pursue your goals.

We see this mindset in almost all stories of success, especially in professional athletes. A challenge arises, doubt attempts to creep in, and the individual decides to persevere. They don't let a fall keep them down. Should you falter, recognize it, learn from it. Notice what doesn't serve you and move forward.

Think of it this way. When you die, will you look back at this moment as well lived? Will you perceive the feelings and thoughts you have, right now, as worth the precious moment of life you gave it? Every moment, every thought you have is giving life. It is growing a perspective. By directing your focus, you are directing your life.

Five

EMOTIONAL CONNECTION

Feel It Out

Remember what it means to be all in? Your thoughts, actions, and emotions are aligned. Essentially, you are present and want what you are doing, when you are doing it. There is no internal disconnect. You are fully committed and response-able. On the journey toward conditioning the mind, at a certain point you have to get out of your head and feel your way there.

The last component, emotion, ties the entire experience together. It connects the thoughts of the mind to the actions of the body, infusing life with the sensations of living. Emotions color experience. Someone who is living all in enjoys fitness. They revel in the feeling of wellness. Delighting in the action, they seek more. They live in harmony with it. The full realization is experiencing the emotion. The manifestation of being all in.

This is when being all in becomes fully integrated. Training your mindset gives you a clear path of potential and fertile soil from which new experiences can grow. Creating meaningful goals focuses and cements the vision. Turning potential into energy, into an experience, takes a certain emotional state. How action is taken, from which place, is just as important (if not more) than the action itself.

Knowing what you now know, it is time to fully integrate your training. The practice includes creating and maintaining an emotional state. However, you have to feel it out for yourself. The desire has to feel good. The process has to feel good. Sometimes it may take a fair amount of self-talk to get to that point. Or the opposite, perhaps you can zone into the feeling easier without thinking about it. Only you can gauge what will work for you at any given moment. There is no one-size-fits-all prescription.

Feel your way there. To do this, presence is required. You have to be response-able, focused, and in tune with your body, mind, and emotions. The more you practice it, the easier it becomes. As awareness increases, so does your ability to deliberately guide the experience.

Start by wetting your appetite. When you go to exercise, focus on intentionally generating an emotional state. Do it for only as long as you can sustain or grow the feeling. Basically, do it as long as it feels good. If it starts to wane or seem overly forced, ease up. It must come from a gentle, simple place before it can be amplified and maintained. Be honest with yourself. If you can only sustain it for a quarter-mile walk, that is fine. The practice is not on the distance you run or weight you lift. It isn't even on the time. The practice is on how you feel leading up to and while taking the action. Practicing the state fans the desire. Tomorrow, maybe even later that day, you will crave more.

As this becomes your training, the body will begin to surprise you. It will feel invigorated and joyously respond with more. Going farther, faster, becoming stronger, more agile. As the mind recognizes this, it will become increasingly instilled in you. The feeling becomes easier to generate from within. Your expectations will rise, and your life will change.

Potential Energy

What is the difference between a pot of water boiling and water standing still? It's temperature. Water does not boil at 211 degrees. It has to be at 212 degrees. That one degree makes all the difference. Granted, there is a build up to that point, but that final degree is transformative. So what is your degree of difference? What sparks in you the difference between sitting on a couch in lethargy and getting up to take action?

The moment when you tune into your feelings and aspire to feel just a little bit better, desire a little more energy, clarity, vigor, fun. When you become present and make the decision to elevate your emotional state, a desire is ignited. That decision, that desire, sweeps across your mind like a fire clearing a field. That moment of awareness is when you turn on the heat. You decide to crank up your emotional state. Emotions are one step away from action. Just as a one-degree increase makes a difference for the water, it makes all the difference for you.

There is a lot of science behind how energy and force are generated and the mechanics of the cooking pot, or your body. At the simplest level, the water would not boil unless the heat was provided. And you would not move unless the emotional experience or desire was present.

You can get aligned action through focusing on your feelings. What does that mean? If you are not feeling inspired, if you are not feeling vitality, focus your attention on generating those emotions. Because that is what it means to get in touch with it—literally to touch or feel that state of being.

So, if you're sitting on the couch thinking about how you want to run but just don't feel like it, recognize what that means. It signifies that right now, with your current state of being, you are not thinking thoughts and feeling emotions that generate the response you desire. What do you do? Wait around for someone to drag you out the door, or for a personal trainer to burst into your home and try to pump you up with enthusiasm? Sure, you could, but you would be waiting quite a while. Moreover, you would be evading responsibility for your life! Remember, only you can decide how to respond. Be response-able! Get in your power, in the moment, and intend to generate the feeling you desire. One step at a time. You most likely will not go from a practiced state of boredom to overjoyed instantaneously.

But you can turn up the heat one degree. Intentionally increase rejuvenation and energy. Then, take the action. One of the best ways to do this is by deliberately creating the atmosphere. After all, contemplating the benefits of working out won't get you off the couch, but an emotion will.

Atmosphere

You create the atmosphere for a party so guests are inclined to feel a certain way and then act a certain way. You set the tone. Create the mood. Creative artists know that when they intentionally set a time to be creative, they focus on their environment and their mentality. They have to prepare themselves in order to be effective. Before you jump into action, prepare yourself.

For example, before you go for a run, or even put on your sneakers, start creating the atmosphere. It is easy! Put on music that is upbeat with lyrics that celebrate life. It should feel positive and fun. Pick songs that evoke those feelings from you. Simply listen. Keep it on in the background as you ease into it. Know that when you are ready, you will go. When you start to notice your toe tapping, hips swaying, or head bopping, keep feeling it. Now, with that emotion, begin getting ready for your workout. Let that feeling carry you through.

Creating the atmosphere is essential, especially for individuals who desire an action but have yet to feel the energy or emotion to get started. Deliberately setting your mood encourages inspired action. It incites you to get moving and to do it from a joyful place.

The pivotal moment wasn't when you went for the run or workout. It wasn't when you put on your sneakers. It was when you decided you wanted to feel a little more elevated, a little more alive, and a little more inclined to move. You decided to put on some music and gently let it happen. You took the initiative, putting yourself in an environment conducive to producing the desired outcome. Eventually this will lead to associating the action with fun. Remember, don't do it for your health, do it to feel your health.

Get Outside

Get outside! Go for a hike in a park, play tennis, practice yoga. Do whatever activity you prefer, and do it outside whenever possible.

Why nature? Because nature reminds us of the beauty of life. It is miraculous. It is vitality. Look around you and appreciate, marvel, and revel. Allow those emotions to stir, even if they are being projected outwardly. This will help ignite the spark within you and familiarize you with those emotional states. Ideally you should do this while moving your body. However, simply sitting outside and practicing this disposition will help. Those emotions are at the foundation of your new perspective. That way of being is the cornerstone of living all in.

While you appear to be appreciating the flow of life in that which is outside of you, in the deepest sense, it is not external. We get so caught up in houses, cars, offices, and technology, that we forget we are part of the nature of this planet. The same miracle that causes the caterpillar to transform into a butterfly, that cracks the seed for the tree to grow, and that causes the sun to rise every morning, is the same life that brought you into this body. So while you think you're appreciating external nature, in the deepest sense you are appreciating life in general. You are admiring the same beauty and vitality that exists within you.

Look for little ways to increase your exposure to nature and this perspective. When taking out the trash, use those steps as a way to witness the miracle of life through the nature around you. Even someone living in a city with sparse trees or plants can look up at the sky. There is always something in nature to help facilitate those feelings. You just have to keep your eyes open to see it.

Daniella's Story

If only you knew what I know. I did not appreciate fitness until something happened. Slowly a new perspective began to emerge within my mind. I didn't cut it down like an unwelcome weed. I cradled it. I kept it secret. I nurtured it, and it grew.

As a child, I enjoyed playing outside in nature. Hiking, riding my bike, whatever outdoor activity it was, there was something grounding in the experience. Yet as a young adult, those activities faded.

Feeling sluggish and discouraged about the circumstances of my life, I went back to what brought me joy as a child. I went to a nearby park to meander, in an attempt to find joy. Meander I did, for quite a while over a couple of visits.

On the park site was a horse ranch. One day I took a moment to simply look at the horses and admire them.

Just then, a horse started galloping for no particular reason. It appeared to be having a lot of fun just galloping about. The horse wasn't running from or to anything. It just felt like moving. It was as if the horse was showing me the joys of living that I had become somewhat oblivious to. The joy of being in a body and experiencing vitality. Well, maybe I could just feel good? Maybe I just felt like running? Maybe I didn't need a reason? At that moment, I decided next time I would bring my sneakers and jog, if only for a minute.

That is exactly what I did. I put on my grungy old sneakers, a T-shirt, and sweats. I picked a short trail in the woods that few people traveled. It didn't matter what I looked like, how fast, or how much I was running. All that mattered was that I felt good about what I was doing, when I was doing it. The first day I didn't run very far, but no one was around for me to care. My distance, my time, the amount of sweat dripping down my face . . . were all my little secret. This became my ritual.

A few visits later, I progressed around the corner of my first mile with ease and enjoyment. In the clearing above, against the blue sky, I saw a flock of birds flying. We have a tendency to admire birds. We look up at them and imagine what it would be like to fly, to feel free and invigorated. Moving gracefully, they glide on the current of some invisible force. At that moment I wondered, what if the birds are looking down at me and imagining what it would be like to run? That is when my perspective blossomed.

This is how we should move. This is how we should live. This is how we should approach our bodies and the blessed physical experiences they bring us.

Made in United States
Orlando, FL
08 April 2023

31890842R00050